C000178294

# The Affordable Keto Diet Recipe Collection

Cheap and Tasty Keto Recipes to Boost Your Meals and Save Your Money

Gerard Short

## © Copyright 2020 - All rights reserved.

The content contained within this book may not be reproduced, duplicated or transmitted without direct written permission from the author or the publisher.

Under no circumstances will any blame or legal responsibility be held against the publisher, or author, for any damages, reparation, or monetary loss due to the information contained within this book. Either directly or indirectly.

**Legal Notice:**

This book is copyright protected. This book is only for personal use. You cannot amend, distribute, sell, use, quote or paraphrase any part, or the content within this book, without the consent of the author or publisher.

**Disclaimer Notice:**

Please note the information contained within this document is for educational and entertainment purposes only. All effort has been executed to present accurate, up to date, and reliable, complete information. No warranties of any kind are declared or implied. Readers acknowledge that the author is not engaging in the rendering of legal, financial, medical or professional advice. The content within this book has been derived from various sources. Please consult a licensed professional before attempting any techniques outlined in this book.

By reading this document, the reader agrees that under no circumstances is the author responsible for any losses, direct or indirect, which are incurred as a result of the use of information contained within this document, including, but not limited to, — errors, omissions, or inaccuracies.

# Table of Contents

# Sicilian-Style Zoodle Spaghetti

Preparation Time : 10 minutes

Cooking time : 15 minutes

Servings : 6

Ingredients

- 4 cups zoodles (spiralled zucchini)
- 2 ounces cubed bacon
- 4 ounces canned sardines, ch opped
- ½ cup canned chopped tomatoes
- 1 tbsp capers
- 1 tbsp parsley
- 1 tsp minced garlic

Directions

1. Pour some of the sardine oil in a pan.
2. Add garlic and cook for 1 minute.
3. Add the bacon and cook for 2 more minutes. Stir in the tomatoes and let simmer for 5 minutes.
4. Add zoodles and sardines and cook for 3 minutes.

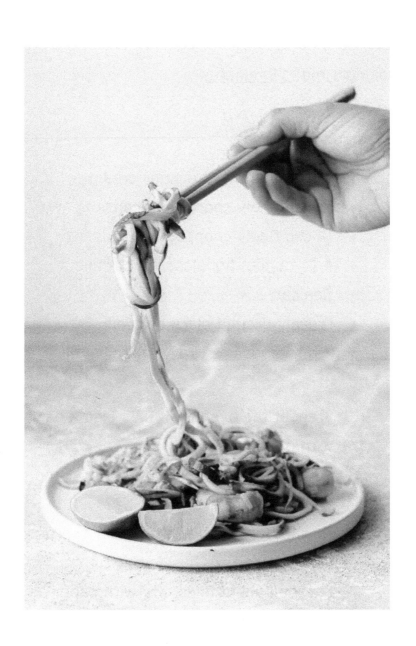

# Baked Nutty Halibut

Preparation Time: 20 minutes

Cooking Time: <u>15 minutes</u>

Servings <u>: 4</u>

Ingredients:

- ½ cup heavy (whipping) cream
- ½ cup finely chopped pecans
- ¼ cup finely chopped almonds
- 4 (4-ounce) boneless halibut fillets
- Sea salt
- Freshly ground black pepper
- 2 tablespoons extra-virgin olive oil

Directions:

1. Preheat the oven to 400°F. Line a baking sheet with parchment.
2. Pour the heavy cream into a bowl and set it on your work surface.
3. In another bowl, stir together the pecans and almonds and set beside the cream.
4. Pat the halibut fillets dry with paper towels and lightly season with salt and pepper.

5. Dip the fillets in the cream, shaking off the excess; then  dredge the fish in the nut mixture so that both sides of each piece are thickly coated.

6. Place the fish on the prepared baking sheet and brush both sides of the pieces generously with olive oil.

7. Bake the fish until the topping is golden and the fish flakes easily with a fork, 12 to 15 minutes. Serve.

8. Make Ahead: The "breaded" fish fillets can be completely put together and then frozen on a baking sheet. Transfer the individual fillets to plastic bags and freeze for up to 1 month. Cook the fillets from frozen, brushed lightly with olive oil, in a 350°F oven for about 35 minutes.

Nutrition:

- Calories 212
- Total Fat: 6.6g
- Carbs: 34.9g
- Sugars: 12.2g
- Protein: 8.9g

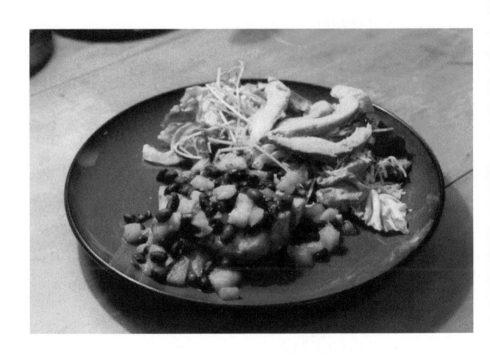

# Sour Cream Salmon with Parmesan

Preparation Time : 10 minutes

Cooking time : 20 minutes

Servings : 6

Ingredients

- 1 cup sour cream
- ½ tbsp minced dill
- ½ lemon, zested and juiced
- Pink salt and black pepper to season
- 4 salmon steaks
- ½ cup grated Parmesan cheese

Directions

1. Preheat oven to 400ºF and line a baking sheet with parchment paper; set aside. In a bowl, mix the sour cream, dill, lemon zest, juice, salt, and black pepper, and set aside.

2. Season the fish with salt and black pepper, drizzle lemon juice on both sides of the fish and arrange them in the baking sheet. Spread the sour cream mixture on each fish  and sprinkle with Parmesan.

3. Bake the fish for 15 minutes and after broil the top for 2 minutes with a close watch for a nice a brown color. Plate the fish and serve with buttery green beans.

Nutrition:

- Calories 251
- Fat 6.2g
- Carbs 44.1g
- Protein 4.2g
- Sugars 3g

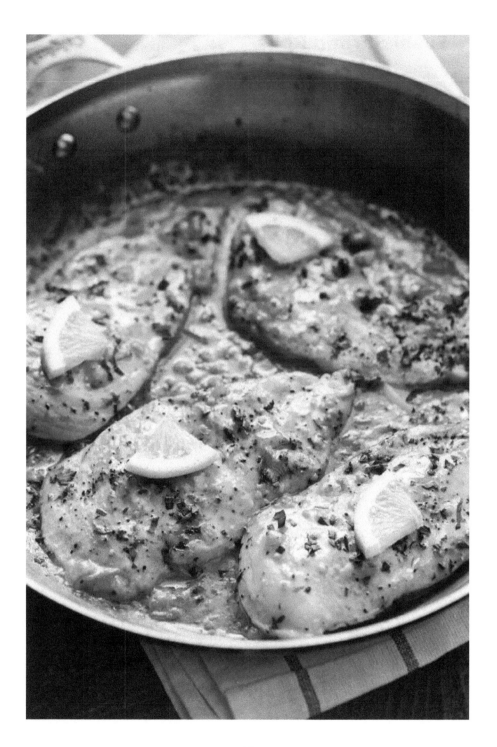

# Sushi Shrimp Rolls

Preparation Time : 10 minutes

Cooking time : 20 minutes

Servings : 6

Ingredients

- 2 cups cooked and chopped shrimp
- 1 tbsp sriracha sauce
- ¼ cucumber, julienned
- 5 hand roll nori sheets
- ¼ cup mayonnaise

Directions

1. Combine shrimp, mayonnaise, cucumber and sriracha sauce in a bowl. Lay out a single nori sheet on a flat surface and spread about 1/5 of the shrimp mixture.
2. Roll the nori sheet as desired.
3. Repeat with the other ingredients. Serve with sugar-free soy sauce.

Nutrition : 233 Calories - 3.3g Fat - 45.8g Carbs - 5.8g Protein - 8.7g Sugars

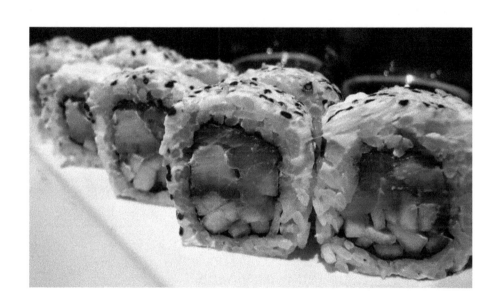

# Grilled Shrimp with Chimichurri Sauce

Preparation Time : 10 minutes

Cooking time : 20 minutes

Servings: 6

Ingredients

- 1 pound shrimp, peeled and deveined
- 2 tbsp olive oil
- Juice of 1 lime
- Chimichurri
- ½ tsp salt
- ¼ cup olive oil
- 2 garlic cloves
- ¼ cup red onions , chopped
- ¼ cup red wine vinegar
- ½ tsp pepper
- 2 cups parsley
- ¼ tsp red pepper flakes

Directions

4. Process the chimichurri ingredients in a blender until smooth; set aside.

5. Combine shrimp, olive oil, and lime juice, in a bowl, and let marinate in the fridge for 30 minutes.
6. Preheat your grill to medium. Add shrimp and cook about 2 minutes per side. Serve shrimp drizzled with the chimichurri sauce.

Nutrition:

- Calories 194
- Fat 5.4g
- Carbs 29.9g
- Protein 8g
- Sugars 5.1g

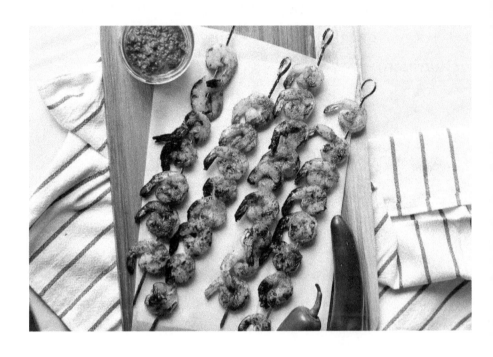

# Coconut Crab Patties

Preparation Time: <u>10 minutes</u>

<u>Cooking time</u> : 50 minutes

Servings <u>: 6</u>

Ingredients

- 2 tbsp coconut oil
- 1 tbsp lemon juice
- 1 cup lump crab meat
- 2 tsp Dijon mustard
- 1 egg, beaten
- 1 ½ tbsp coconut flour

Directions

1. In a bowl to the crabmeat, add all the ingredients, except for the oil; mix well to combine.
2. Make patties out of the mixture. Melt the coconut oil in a skillet over medium heat. Add the crab patties and cook for about 2-3 minutes per side.

<u>Nutrition</u> : Calories 277 - Fat 26.2g - Carbs 9g - Sugar 4g - Protein 7.5g – Cholesterol 31mg

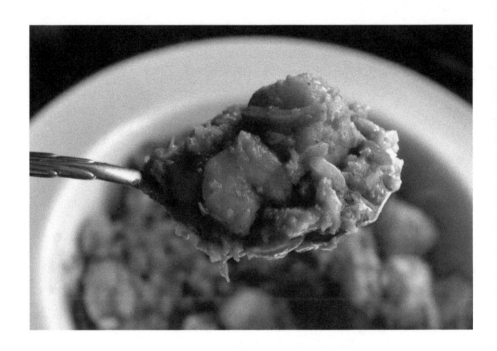

# Shrimp in Curry Sauce

Preparation Time : 10 minutes

Cooking time : 20 minutes

Servings : 6

Ingredients

- ½ ounce grated Parmesan cheese
- 1 egg, beaten
- ¼ tsp curry powder
- 2 tsp almond flour
- 12 shrimp, shelled
- 3 tbsp coconut oil
- Sauce
- 2 tbsp curry leaves
- 2 tbsp butter
- ½ onion, diced
- ½ cup heavy cream
- ½ ounce cheddar cheese, shredded

Directions

1. Combine all dry ingredients for the batter.
2. Melt the coconut oil in a skillet over medium heat. Dip the shrimp in the egg first, and then

coat with the dry mixture. Fry until golden and crispy.

3. In another skillet, melt butter.
4. Add onion and cook for 3 minutes.
5. Add curry leaves and cook for 30 seconds. Stir in heavy cream and cheddar and cook until thickened.
6. Add shrimp and coat well.
7. Serve.

Nutrition:

- Calories 190
- Fat 16.3 g
- Carbohydrates 2.3 g
- Sugar 0.2 g
- Protein 8.7 g
- Cholesterol 52 mg

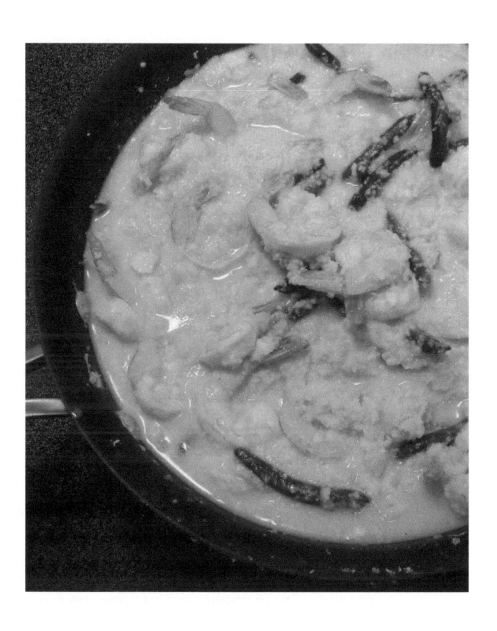

# Tilapia with Olives & Tomato Sauce

Preparation Time: <u>10 minutes</u>

Cooking time: <u>50 minutes</u>

Servings <u>: 6</u>

Ingredients

- 4 tilapia fillets
- 2 garlic cloves, minced
- 2 tsp oregano
- 14 ounces diced tomatoes
- 1 tbsp olive oil
- ½ red onion, chopped
- 2 tbsp parsley
- ¼ cup kalamata olives

Directions

1. Heat olive oil in a skillet over medium heat and cook the onion for 3 minutes.
2. Add garlic and oregano and cook for 30 seconds. Stir in tomatoes and bring the mixture to a boil. Reduce the heat and simmer for 5 minutes.
3. Add olives and tilapia and cook for about 8 minutes.

4. Serve the tilapia with tomato sauce.

Nutrition:

- Calories 66
- Fat 3.3 g
- Carbohydrates 9.9 g
- Sugar 5.1 g
- Protein 0.8 g
- Cholesterol 9 mg

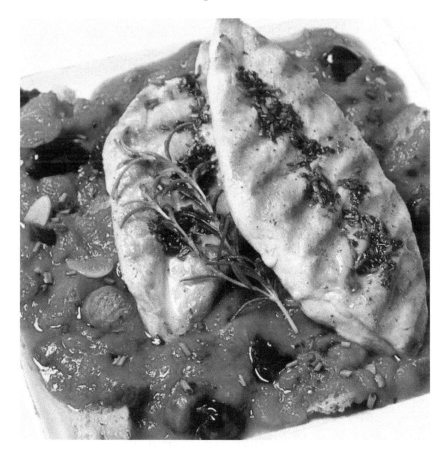

# Lemon Garlic Shrimp

Preparation Time: <u>10 minutes</u>

<u>Cooking time</u> : 50 minutes

Servings <u>: 6</u>

Ingredients

- ½ cup butter, divided
- 2 lb. shrimp, peeled and deveined
- Salt and black pepper to taste
- ¼ tsp sweet paprika
- 1 tbsp minced garlic
- 3 tbsp water
- 1 lemon, zested and juiced
- 2 tbsp chopped parsley

Directions

1. Melt half of the butter in a large skillet over medium heat, season the shrimp with salt, black pepper, paprika, and add to the butter.
2. Stir in the garlic and cook the shrimp for 4 minutes on both sides until pink. Remove to a bowl and set aside.
3. Put the remaining butter in the skillet; include the lemon zest, juice, and water.

4. Add the shrimp, parsley, and adjust the taste with salt and  pepper.

5. Cook for 2 minutes.

6. Serve shrimp and sauce with squash pasta.

Nutrition:

- Calories 245
- Fat 7.5 g
- Carbohydrates 32.8 g
- Sugar 3.5 g
- Protein 11.8 g
- Cholesterol 22 mg

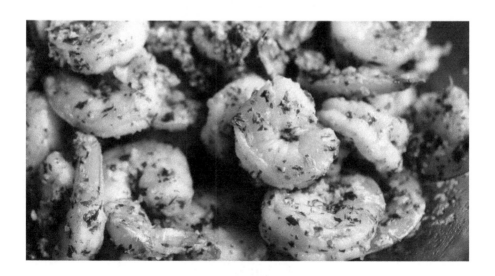

# Seared Scallops with Chorizo and Asiago Cheese

Preparation Time: <u>10 minutes</u>

<u>Cooking time</u> : 30 minutes

Servings <u>: 6</u>

Ingredients

- 2 tbsp ghee
- 16 fresh scallops
- 8 ounces chorizo, chopped
- 1 red bell pepper, seeds removed, sliced
- 1 cup red onions, finely chopped
- 1 cup asiago cheese, grated
- Salt and black pepper to taste

Directions

1. Melt half of the ghee in a skillet over medium heat and cook the onion and bell pepper for 5 minutes until tender.
2. Add the chorizo and stir-fry for another 3 minutes. Remove and set aside.
3. Pat dry the scallops with paper towels, and season with salt and pepper.

4. Add the remaining ghee to the skillet and sear the scallops for 2 minutes on each side to have a golden-brown color.
5. Add the chorizo mixture back and warm through. Transfer to serving platter and top with asiago cheese.

Nutrition:

- Calories 78
- Fat 4.9 g
- Carbohydrates 8.5 g
- Sugar 4.4 g
- Protein 2 g
- Cholesterol 0 mg

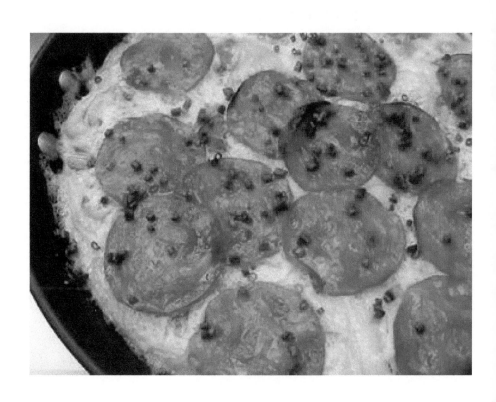

# Tuna Cakes

Preparation Time: <u>10 minutes</u>

Cooking time: <u>10 minute s</u>

Servings <u>: 12</u>

Ingredients:

- 15 ounces canned tuna, drained well and flaked
- 2 eggs
- ½ teaspoon dried dill
- 1 teaspoon dried parsley
- ½ cup onion chopped
- 1 teaspoon garlic powder
- Salt and ground black pepper, to taste
- Oil, for frying

Directions <u>:</u>

1. In a bowl, mix tuna with salt, pepper, dill, parsley, onion, garlic powder, eggs, and stir well.
2. Shape tuna cakes and place on a plate.
3. Heat a pan with oil over medium–high heat, add tuna cakes, cook for 5 minutes on each side. Divide on plates and serve.

Nutrition:

- Calories 322
- Fat 7.8 g
- Carbohydrates 44.3 g
- Sugar 7.3 g
- Protein 20.7 g
- Cholesterol 13 mg

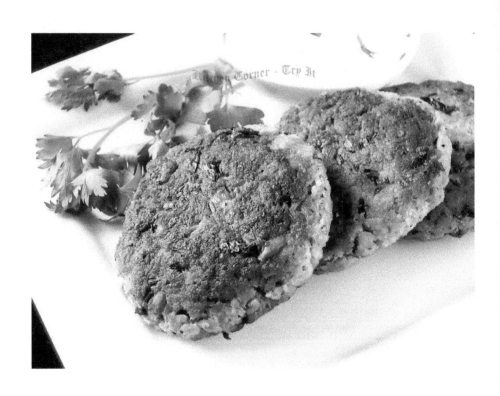

# Pan-roasted Cod

Preparation Time: <u>10 minutes</u>

<u>Cooking time</u> : 20 minutes

Servings <u>: 4</u>

Ingredients <u>:</u>

- 1-pound cod, cut into medium–sized pieces
- Salt and ground black pepper, to t aste
- 2 green onions, chopped
- 2 garlic cloves, peeled and minced
- 2 tablespoons soy sauce
- 1 cup fish stock
- 1 tablespoon balsamic vinegar
- 1 tablespoon fresh ginger, grated
- ½ teaspoon red chili flakes

Directions <u>:</u>

1. Heat a pan over medium–high heat, add fish pieces, and brown on each side.
2. Add garlic, green onions, salt, pepper, soy sauce, fish stock, vinegar, chili pepper, ginger, stir, cover, reduce heat, and cook for 20 minutes.
3. Divide on plates and serve.

Nutrition:

- Calories 142
- Fat 5.9 g
- Carbohydrates 17 g
- Sugar 2.2 g
- Protein 6.3 g
- Cholesterol 0 mg

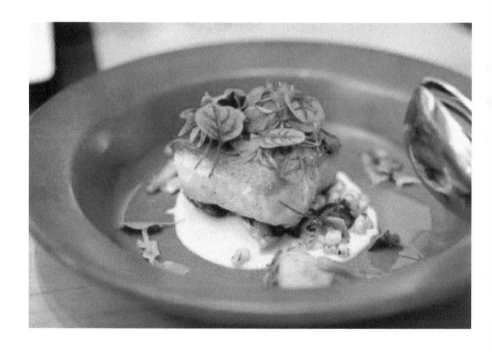

# Sea Bass with Capers

Preparation Time: <u>10 minutes</u>

Cooking time: <u>15 minutes</u>

Servings <u>: 4</u>

Ingredients:

- 1 lemon, sliced
- 1-pound sea bass fillet
- 2 tablespoons capers
- 2 tablespoons fresh dill
- Salt and ground black pepper, to taste

Directions :

1. Put sea bass fillet into a baking dish, season with salt, and pepper, add capers, dill, and lemon slices on top.
2. Place in an oven at 350ºF and bake for 15 minutes.

Nutrition:

- Calories 55
- Fat 0.4 g
- Carbohydrates 11.6 g
- Sugar 5 g
- Protein 3.4 g

- Cholesterol 0 mg

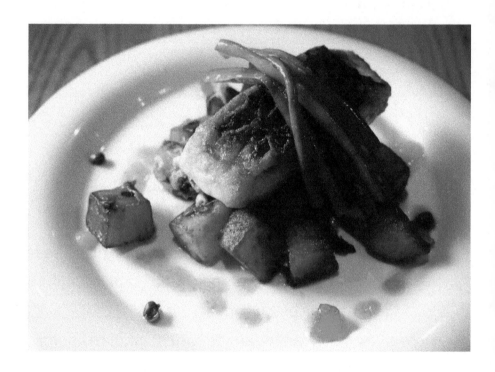

# Cod with Arugula

Preparation Time : 10 minutes

Cooking time : 20 minutes

Servings : 4

Ingredients :

- 2 cod fillets
- 1 tablespoon olive oil
- Salt and ground black pepper, to taste
- Juice of 1 lemon
- cup arugula
- ½ cup black olives, pitted and sliced
- 2 tablespoons capers
- 1 garlic clove, peeled and chopped

Directions :

1. Arrange fish fillets in a heatproof dish, season with salt, pepper, drizzle the oil and lemon juice, toss to coat, place in an oven at 450ºF, and bake for 20 minutes.
2. In a food processor, mix arugula with salt, pepper, capers, olives, garlic, and blend well.
3. Arrange the fish on plates, top with arugula tapenade, and serve.

Nutrition:

- Calories 240
- Total Fats 12g
- Carbs: 12g
- Protein 28g
- Dietary Fiber: 2.5g

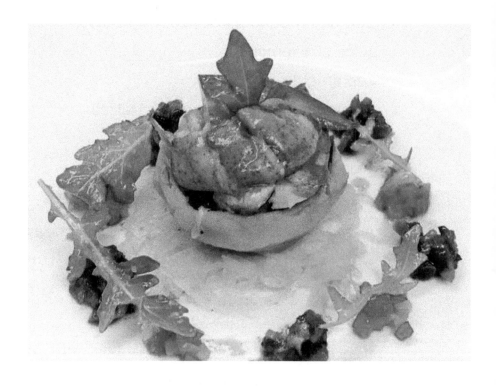

# Baked Halibut with Vegetables

Preparation Time: <u>10 minutes</u>

Cooking time: <u>35 minutes</u>

Servings <u>: 4</u>

Ingredients:

- 1 red bell pepper, seeded and chopped
- 1 yellow bell pepper, seeded and chopped
- 1 teaspoon balsamic vinegar
- 1 tablespoon olive oil
- 2 halibut fillets
- 2 cups baby spinach
- Salt and ground black pepper, to taste
- 1 teaspoon cumin

Directions <u>:</u>

1. In a bowl, mix bell peppers with salt, pepper, half of the oil, and vinegar, toss to coat well, and transfer to a baking dish.
2. Place in oven at 400ºF and bake for 20 minutes.
3. Heat a pan with the rest of the oil over medium heat, add fish, season with salt, pepper, cumin, and brown on all sides.

4. Take baking dish out of the oven, add the spinach, stir gently, and divide the whole mixture on plates.

5. Add fish on the side, sprinkle with salt and pepper, and serve.

Nutrition:

- Calories 240
- Total Fats 0.2g
- Carbs: 9g
- Protein 20g
- Dietary Fiber: 2g

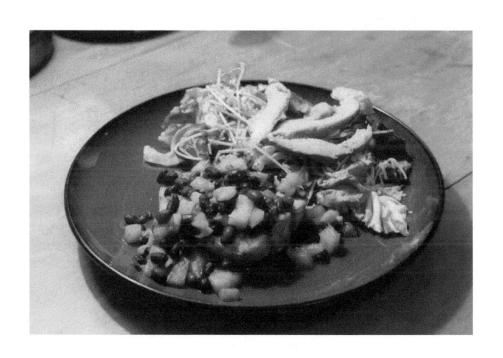

# Fish Curry

Preparation Time : 10 minutes

Cooking time: 25 minutes

Servings : 4

Ingredients :

- 4 white fish fillets
- ½ teaspoon mustard seeds
- Salt and ground black pepper, to taste
- 2 green chilies, chopped
- 1 teaspoon fresh ginger, grated
- 1 teaspoon curry powder
- ¼ teaspoon cumin
- tablespoons coconut oil
- 1 onion, peeled and chopped
- 1-inch turmeric root, grated
- ¼ cup fresh cilantro
- 1½ cups coconut cream
- garlic cloves, peeled and minced

Directions :

1. Heat a saucepan with half of the coconut oil over medium heat, add mustard seeds, and cook for 2 minutes.

2. Add ginger, onion, garlic, stir, and cook for 5 minutes. Add turmeric, curry powder, chilies, and cumin, stir, and cook for 5 minutes.
3. Add coconut milk, salt, and pepper, stir, bring to a boil, and cook for 15 minutes.
4. Heat another pan with remaining oil over medium heat, add fish, stir, and cook for 3 minutes.
5. Add to curry sauce, stir, and cook for 5 minutes.
6. Add cilantro, stir, divide into bowls, and serve.

Nutrition:

- Calories 240
- Total Fats 0.2g
- Carbs: 9g
- Protein 20g
- Dietary Fiber: 2g

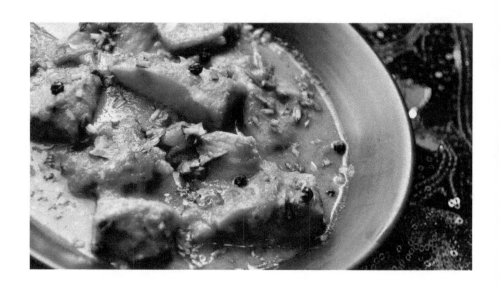

# Keto Baked Tilapia with Cherry Tomatoes

Preparation Time : 10 minutes

Cooking time: 25 minutes

Servings : 4

Ingredients Needed :

- Butter (2 tsp.)
- Tilapia fillets (2 - 4 oz. each)
- Cherry tomatoes (8)
- Pitted black olives (.25 cup)
- Salt (.5 tsp.)
- Paprika (.25 tsp.)
- Black pepper (.25 tsp.)
- Garlic powder (1 tsp.)
- Lemon juice (1 tbsp.)
- Optional: Balsamic vinegar (1 tbsp.)

Directions

1. Warm the oven to reach 375º F.
2. Grease a roasting pan and add the butter along with the olives and tomatoes.
3. Season the tilapia with the spices. Squeeze the lemon and spritz the fish fillets, adding them to the pan.

4. Add a piece of foil over the pan. Bake until the fish easily flakes (25 to 30 min.).

5. Garnish with the vinegar if desired.

Nutrition:

- Calories 84
- Fat 2.1 g
- Carbohydrates 14.7 g
- Sugar 3.2 g
- Protein 3.3 g
- Cholesterol 5 mg

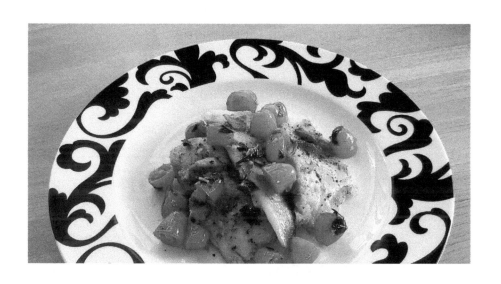

# Green Coconut Smoothie

Preparation Time: <u>10 minutes</u>

Servings : <u>3</u>

Ingredients :

- 1 1/4 cup coconut milk canned
- 2 Tablespoon chia seeds
- 1 cup of fresh kale leaves
- 1 cup of spinach leaves
- 1 scoop vanilla protein powder
- 1 cup of ice cubes
- Granulated stevia sweetener to taste; optional
- 1/2 cup water

Directions :

1. Rinse and clean kale and the spinach leaves from any dirt.
2. Add all ingredients in your blender.
3. Blend until you get a nice smoothie.
4. Serve into chilled glass.

Nutrition:

- Calories 323
- Total Fats 9.6g
- Carbs: 59.7g
- Protein 9.2g

- Dietary Fiber: 10.6g

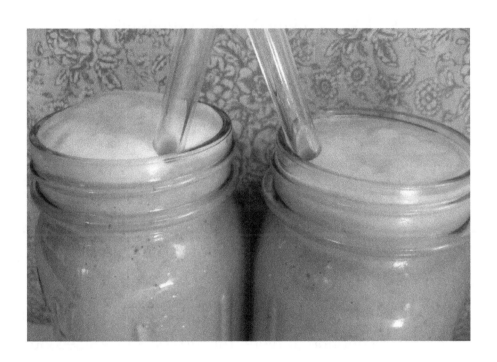

# Instant Coffee Smoothie

Preparation Time : 20 minutes

Servings: 3

Ingredients :

- 2 cups of instant coffee
- 1 cup almond milk or coconut milk
- 1/4 cup heavy cream
- 2 Tablespoon cocoa powder unsweetened
- 1 - 2 Handful of fresh spinach leaves
- 10 drops liquid stevia

Directions :

1. Make a coffee; set aside.
2. Place all remaining ingredients in your fast-speed blender; blend for 45 - 60 seconds or until done.
3. Pour your instant coffee in a blender and continue to blend for further 30 - 45 seconds.
4. Serve immediately.

Nutrition:

- Calories 338
- Total Fats 29.2g
- Carbs: 18.1g
- Protein 8.8g

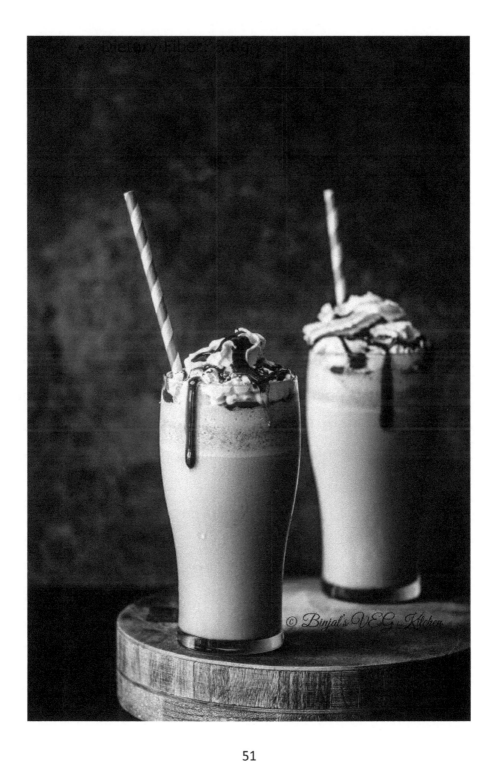

© Binjal's VEG Kitchen

# Keto Blood Sugar Adjuster Smoothie

Preparation Time: <u>10 minutes</u>

Servings: <u>3</u>

Ingredients :

- 2 cups of green cabbage
- 1/2 avocado
- 1 Tablespoon Apple cider vinegar
- Juice of 1 lemon
- 1 cup of water
- 1 cup of crushed ice cubes for serving

Directions :

1. Place all ingredients in your high-speed blender or in a food processor and blend until smooth and soft. Serve in chilled glasses with crushed ice.

<u>Nutrition</u> : Kcal 243 - Carbs 61g - Fat 1g - Protein 2g

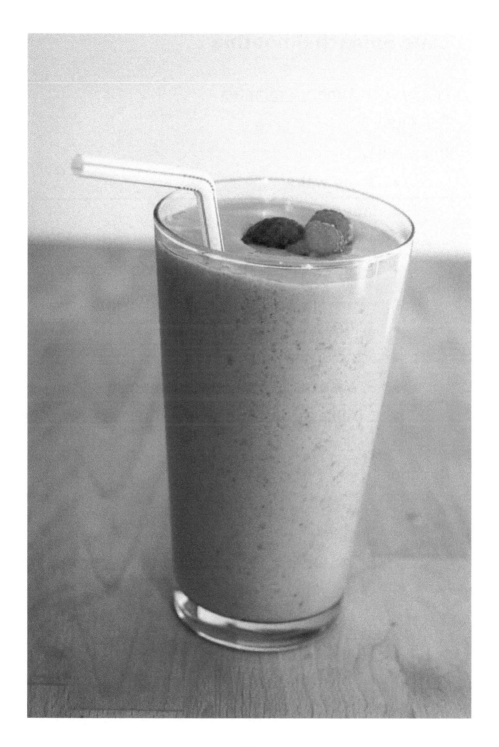

# Lime Spinach Smoothie

Preparation Time : 5 minutes

Servings: 3

Ingredients:

- 1 cup water
- lime juice 1-2 limes
- 1 green apple cut into chunks; core discarded
- 2 cups fresh spinach, roughly chopped
- 1/2 cup fresh chopped fresh mint
- 1/2 avocado
- Ice crushed
- 1/4 teaspoon ground cinnamon
- 1 Tablespoon natural sweetener of your choice optional

Directions :

1. Place all ingredients in your high-speed blender.
2. Blend for 45 - 60 seconds or until your smoothie is smooth and creamy.
3. Serve in a chilled glass.
4. Adjust sweetener to taste.

Nutrition:

- Kcal 202

- Carbs 23g
- Fat 10g
- Protein 9g

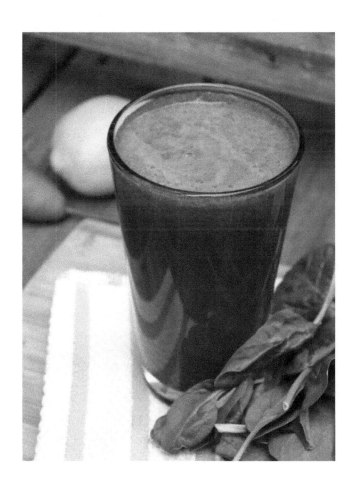

# Protein Coconut Smoothie

Preparation Time : 15 minutes

Servings: 3

Ingredients :

- 1 1/2 cup of coconut milk canned
- 1 cup of fresh spinach finely chopped
- 1 scoop vanilla protein powder
- 2 Tablespoon chia seeds
- 1 cup of ice cubes crushed
- 2 - 3 Tablespoon Stevia granulated natural sweetener optional

Directions :

1. Rinse and clean your spinach leaves from any dirt.
2. Place all ingredients from the list above in a blender.
3. Blend until you get a smoothie like consistently.
4. Serve into chilled glass and it is ready to drink.

Nutrition: Kcal 287 - Carbs 22g - Fat 14g - Protein 17g

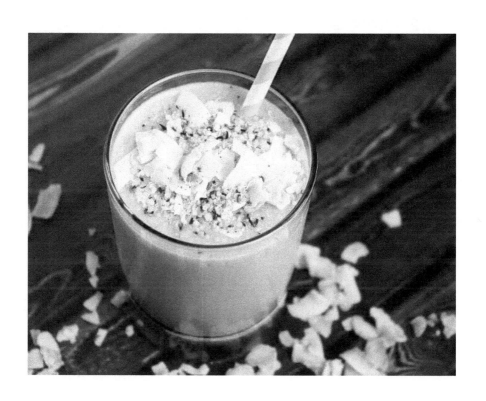

# Strong Spinach and Hemp Smoothie

Preparation Time : 10 minutes

Servings : 3

Ingredients :

- 1 cup almond milk
- 1 small ripe banana
- 2 Tablespoon hemp seeds
- 2 handful fresh spinach leaves
- 1 teaspoon pure vanilla extract
- 1 cup of water
- 2 Tablespoon of natural sweetener such Stevia, Truvia...etc.

Directions :

1. First, rinse and clean your spinach leaves from any dirt.
2. Place the spinach in a blender or food processor along with remaining ingredients.
3. Blend for 45 - 60 seconds or until done.
4. Add more or less sweetener.
5. Serve.

Nutrition : Kcal 229 - Carbs 20g - Fat 15g - Protein 9g

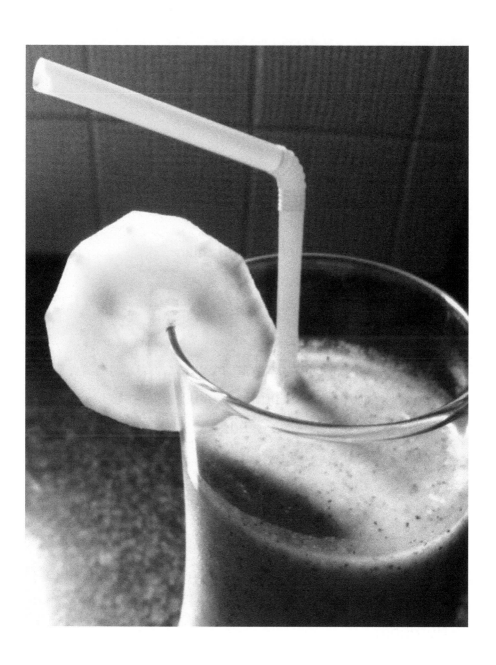

# Green Low Carb Breakfast Smoothie

Preparation Time: <u>5 minutes</u>

Servings <u>: 3</u>

Ingredients <u>:</u>

- 1 oz of spinach
- 2 oz of celery
- 1 ½ cups of almond milk
- 2 oz avocado
- 2 oz of cucumber
- 1 tbsp coconut oil
- 1 scoop of protein powder
- 10 drops of liquid stevia
- ½ tsp of chia seeds

Directions <u>:</u>

1. Add almond milk and spinach to blender.
2. Blend briefly.
3. Add the rest of the ingredients
4. Pour mixture into a glass and sprinkle chia seeds on top.

Nutrition:

- Kcal 276
- Carbs 25g
- Fat 18

- Protein 9g

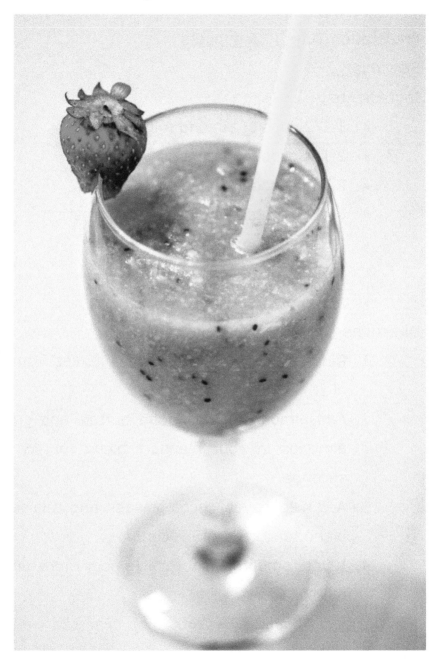

# Total Almond Smoothie

Preparation Time : 15 minutes

Servings : 3

Ingredients :

- 1 1/2 cups of almond milk
- 2 Tablespoon of almond butter
- 2 Tablespoon ground almonds
- 1 cup of fresh kale leaves or to taste
- 1/2 teaspoon of cocoa powder
- 1 Tablespoon chia seeds
- 1/2 cup of water

Directions :

1. Rinse and carefully clean kale leaves from any dirt.
2. Add almond milk, almond butter, and ground almonds in your blender; blend for 45 - 60 seconds.
3. Add kale leaves, cocoa powder, and chia seeds; blend for further 45 seconds.
4. If your smoothie is too thick, pour more almond milk or water.

Nutrition : Kcal 377 - Carbs 37g - Fat 12g - Protein 31g

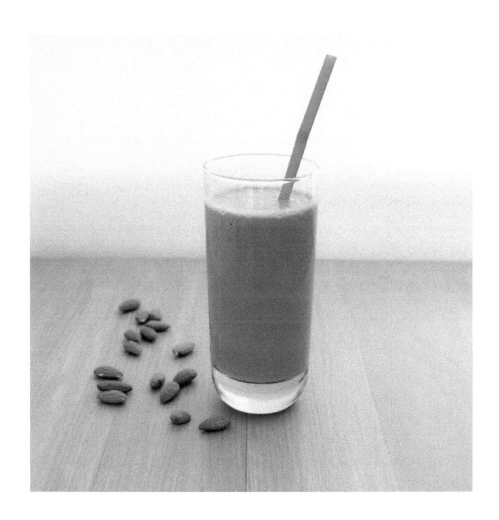

# Ultimate Green Mix Smoothie

Preparation Time: <u>15 minutes</u>

Servings : <u>3</u>

Ingredients :

- Handful of spinach leaves
- Handful of collards greens
- Handful of lettuce, cos or romain
- 1 1/2 cup of almond milk
- 1/2 cup of water
- 1/4 cup of stevia granulated sweetener
- 1 teaspoon pure vanilla extract
- 1 cup crushed ice cubes optional

Directions :

1. Rinse and carefully clean your greens from any dirt.
2. Place all ingredients from the list above in your blender or food processor.
3. Blend until done or 45 - 30 seconds.
4. Serve with or without crushed ice.

Nutrition:

- Kcal 315
- Carbs 17g
- Fat 12g

- Protein 26g

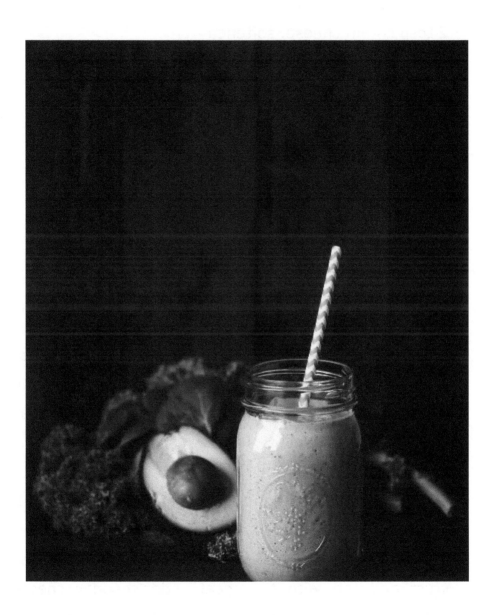

# Taco Beef Pizza

## Ingredients for 4 servings

1 lb ground beef

2 tbsp cream cheese, softened

2 cups shredded mozzarella

1 egg

¾ cup almond flour

2 tsp taco seasoning

½ cup cheese sauce

1 cup grated cheddar cheese

1 cup chopped lettuce

1 tomato, diced

¼ cup sliced black olives

1 cup sour cream for topping

## Directions and Total Time: approx. 35 minutes

Preheat oven to 3750 F. Line a pizza pan with parchment paper. Microwave the mozzarella and cream cheeses for 1 minute. Remove and mix in egg and almond flour.

Spread the mixture on the pan and bake for 15 minutes. Put the beef in a pot and cook for 5 minutes. Stir in taco seasoning. Spread the cheese sauce on the crust and top with the meat. Add cheddar cheese, lettuce, tomato, and black olives. Bake until the cheese melts, 5 minutes. Remove the pizza, drizzle sour cream on top, and serve.

**Per serving:** Cal 589; Net Carbs 7.9g; Fat 31g; Protein 71g

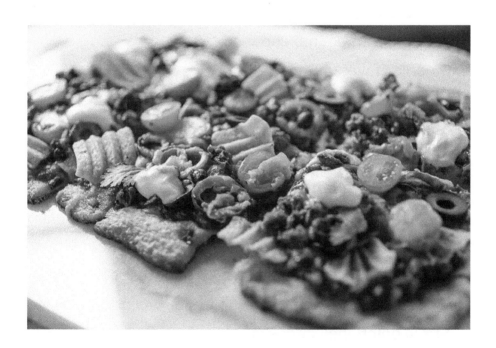

# Cauli Rice with Beef & Cashew Nuts

## Ingredients for 4 servings

1 ½ lb chuck steak, cubed

4 cups cauliflower rice

3 tbsp olive oil

2 large eggs, beaten

1 tbsp avocado oil

1 red onion, finely chopped

½ cup chopped bell peppers

½ cup green beans, chopped

3 garlic cloves, minced

¼ cup coconut aminos

1 cup toasted cashew nuts

1 tbsp toasted sesame seeds

## Directions and Total Time: approx. 25 minutes

Warm 2 tbsp olive oil in a wok over medium heat and cook the beef for 7-8 minutes; set aside. Pour the eggs in the wok and scramble for 2-3 minutes; set aside.

Add the remaining olive oil and avocado oil to heat. Stir in onion, bell peppers, green beans, and garlic. Sauté until soft, 3 minutes. Pour in cauliflower rice, coconut aminos, and stir until evenly combined.

Mix in the beef, eggs, and cashew nuts and cook for 3 minutes. Dish into serving plates and garnish with sesame seeds. Serve.

**Per serving:** Cal 498; Net Carbs 3.2g; Fat 292; Protein 48g

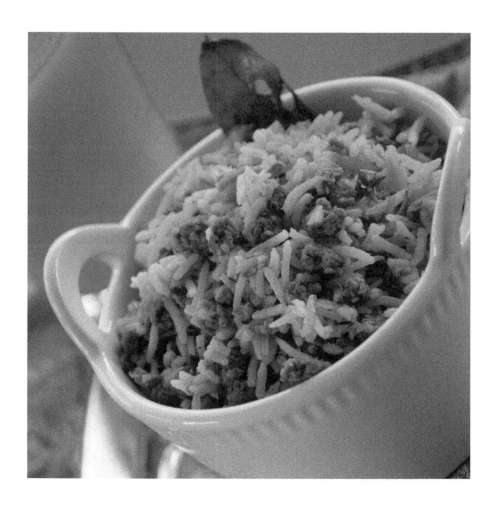

# Grandma´s Meatballs

## Ingredients for 4 servings

1 tbsp olive oil

2 tbsp melted butter

1 lb ground beef

1 red onion, finely chopped

2 red bell peppers, chopped

2 garlic cloves, minced

1 tsp dried basil

2 tbsp tamari sauce

1 tbsp dried rosemary

Salt and black pepper to taste

## Directions and Total Time: approx. 30 minutes

Preheat the oven to 380 F. In a bowl, mix beef, onion, bell peppers, garlic, butter, basil, tamari sauce, salt, pepper, and rosemary. Form 1-inch meatballs from the mixture and place them on a greased baking sheet.

Drizzle olive oil over the beef and bake in the oven for 20 minutes or until the meatballs brown on the outside. Serve topped with ranch dressing.

**Per serving:** Cal 622; Net Carbs 2.5g; Fat 33g; Protein 79g

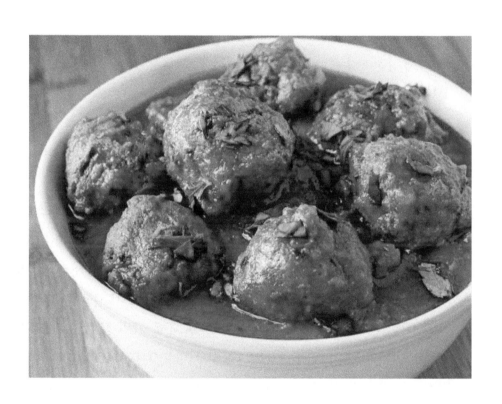

# Beef, Bell Pepper & Mushroom Kebabs

## Ingredients for 4 servings

1 lb cremini mushrooms, halved

2 lb beef tri-tip steak, cubed

2 tbsp coconut oil

2 yellow bell peppers

1 tbsp tamari sauce

1 lime, juiced

1 tbsp ginger powder

½ tsp ground cumin

## Directions and Total Time: approx. 15 min + cooling time

Deseed the bell peppers and cut them into squares. In a bowl, mix coconut oil, tamari sauce, lime juice, ginger, and cumin powder. Add in the beef, mushrooms, and bell peppers; toss to coat. Cover the bowl with plastic wrap and marinate for 1 hour. Preheat the grill to high heat. Take off the plastic wrap and thread the mushrooms, beef, and bell peppers in this order on skewers until the ingredients are exhausted. Grill the skewers for 5 minutes per side. Remove to serving plates and serve warm with steamed cauliflower rice or braised asparagus.

**Per serving:** Cal 379; Net Carbs 3.2g; Fat 23g; Protein 49g

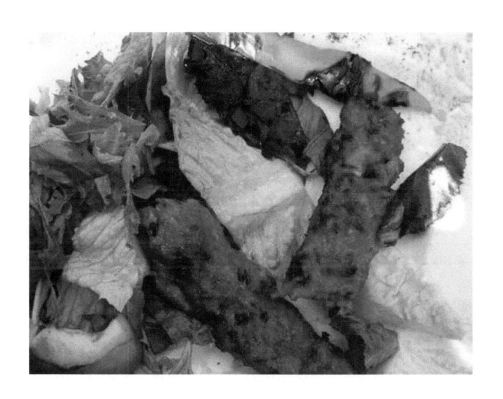

# Mushroom & Beef Stir-Fry
## Ingredients for 4 servings

1 lb shiitake mushrooms, halved

1 lb chuck steak

2 sprigs rosemary, chopped

1 green bell pepper, chopped

4 slices prosciutto, chopped

1 tbsp coconut oil

1 tbsp pureed garlic

## Directions and Total Time: approx. 30 minutes

Using a sharp knife, slice the chuck steak thinly against the grain and cut it into smaller pieces. Heat a skillet over medium heat and cook prosciutto until brown and crispy; set aside. Melt coconut oil in the skillet and cook the beef until brown, 6-8 minutes. Remove to the prosciutto plate. Add mushrooms and bell pepper to the skillet and sauté until softened, 5 minutes. Stir in prosciutto, beef, rosemary, and garlic. Season to taste and cook for 4 minutes. Serve with buttered green beans.

**Per serving:** Cal 229; Net Carbs 2.1g; Fat 12g; Protein 32g

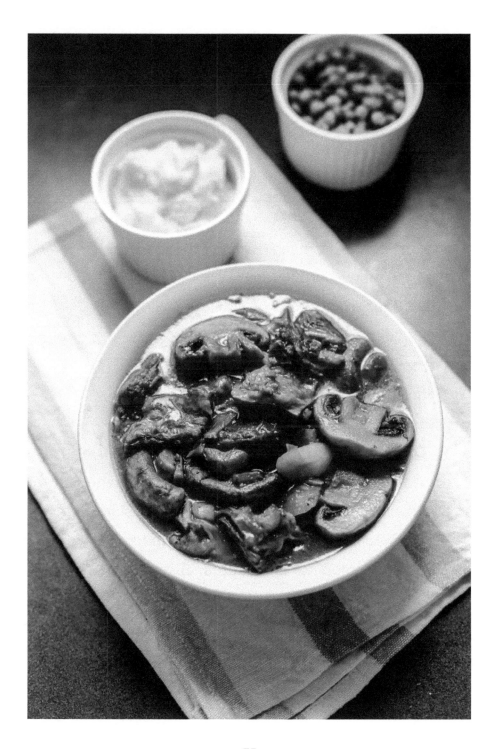

# Asian-Style Creamy Beef
## Ingredients for 4 servings

4 large rib-eye steak

1 green bell pepper, sliced

1 red bell pepper, sliced

2 long red chilies, sliced

2 tbsp ghee

2 garlic cloves, minced

½ cup chopped brown onion

1 cup beef stock

1 cup coconut milk

1 tbsp Thai green curry paste

1 lime, juiced

2 tbsp chopped cilantro

## Directions and Total Time: approx. 40 minutes

Warm the 1 tbsp of ghee in a pan over medium heat and cook the beef for 3 minutes on each side. Remove to a plate. Add the remaining ghee to the skillet and sauté garlic and onion for 3 minutes. Stir-fry in bell peppers and red chili until softened, 5 minutes. Pour in beef stock, coconut milk, curry paste, and lime juice. Let simmer for 4 minutes. Put the beef back into the sauce. Cook for 10 minutes and transfer the pan to the oven. Cook further under the broiler for 5 minutes. Garnish with cilantro and serve with cauliflower rice.

**Per serving:** Cal 638; Net Carbs 2.6g; Fat 35g; Protein 69g

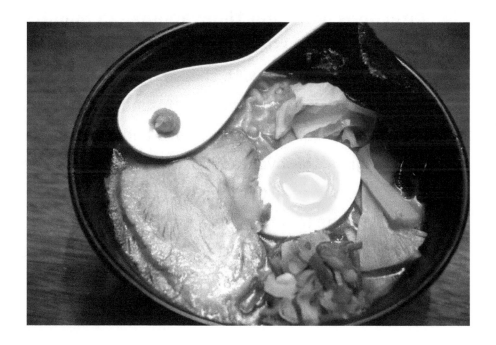

# Beef Hot Dogs in Bacon Wraps
## Ingredients for 4 servings

16 bacon slices

½ cup grated Gruyere cheese

8 large beef hot dogs

1 tsp onion powder

1 tsp garlic powder

Salt and black pepper to taste

### Directions and Total Time: approx. 25 minutes

Preheat oven to 380 F. Cut a slit in the middle of each hot dog and stuff evenly with cheese. Wrap each hot dog with 2 bacon slices and secure with toothpicks. Season with onion and garlic powders, salt, and pepper. Place the hot dogs in the oven and slide in the cookie sheet beneath the rack to catch dripping grease. Cook for 15 minutes until the bacon browns and crisps. Serve.

**Per serving:** Cal 763; Net Carbs 4g; Fat 61g; Protein 42g

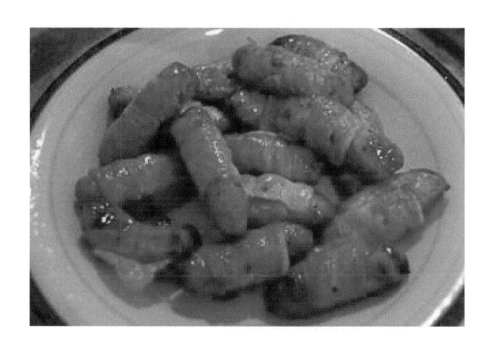

# Jerked Beef Stew
## Ingredients for 4 servings

½ scotch bonnet pepper, chopped

1 onion, chopped

2 tbsp olive oil

1 tsp ginger paste

1 tsp soy sauce

1 lb beef stew meat, cubed

1 red bell pepper, chopped

2 green chilies, chopped

1 cup tomatoes, chopped

1 tbsp fresh cilantro, chopped

1 garlic clove, minced

¼ cup vegetable broth

Salt and black pepper to taste

¼ cup black olives, chopped

1 tsp jerk seasoning

## Directions and Total Time: approx. 80 minutes

Brown the beef on all sides in warm olive oil over medium heat; remove and set aside. Stir-fry in the red bell peppers, green chilies, jerk seasoning, garlic, scotch bonnet pepper, onion, ginger paste, and soy sauce, for about 5-6 minutes. Pour in the tomatoes and broth, and cook for 1 hour. Stir in the olives, adjust the seasonings and serve sprinkled with fresh cilantro.

**Per serving:** Cal 235; Fat 13g; Net Carbs 2.8g; Protein 26g

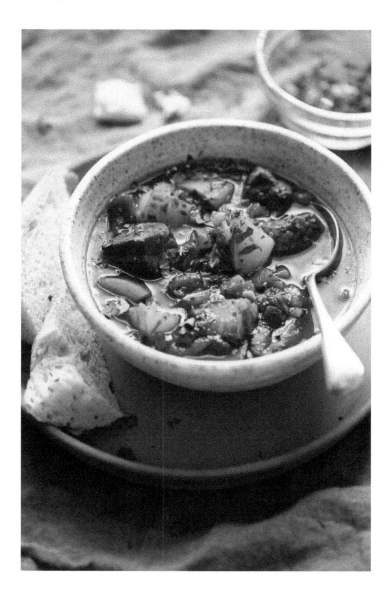

# Coconut-Olive Beef with Mushrooms

## Ingredients for 4 servings

¼ cup button mushrooms, sliced

4 rib-eye steaks

3 tbsp butter

1 yellow onion, chopped

1/3 cup coconut milk

2 tbsp coconut cream

1/2 tsp dried thyme

2 tbsp chopped parsley

3 tbsp black olives, sliced

## Directions and Total Time: approx. 30 minutes

Warm 2 tbsp butter in a deep skillet over medium heat. Add and sauté the mushrooms for 4 minutes until tender. Stir in onion and cook further for 3 minutes; set aside. Melt the remaining butter in the skillet and cook the beef for 10 minutes on both sides. Pour mushrooms and onion back to the skillet and add milk, coconut cream, thyme, and 1 tbsp of parsley. Stir and simmer for 2 minutes. Mix in black olives and turn the heat off. Serve garnished with the remaining parsley.

**Per serving:** Cal 643; Net Carbs 1.9g; Fat 42g; Protein 71g

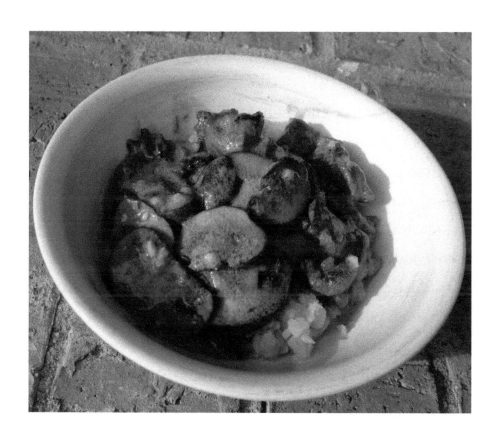

# Cilantro Beef Curry with Cauliflower

## Ingredients for 4 servings

1 head cauliflower, cut into florets

1 tbsp olive oil

½ lb ground beef

1 garlic clove, minced

1 tsp turmeric

1 tbsp cilantro, chopped

1 tbsp ginger paste

½ tsp garam masala

5 oz canned whole tomatoes

Salt and chili pepper to taste

¼ cup water

## Directions and Total Time: approx. 30 minutes

Heat oil in a saucepan over medium heat, add the beef, garlic, ginger paste, and garam masala. Cook for 5 minutes while breaking any lumps. Stir in the tomatoes and cauliflower, season with salt, turmeric, and chili pepper, and cook covered for 6 minutes. Add the water and bring to a boil over medium heat for 10 minutes or until the water has reduced by half. Spoon the curry into serving bowls and serve sprinkled with cilantro.

**Per serving:** Cal 365; Fat 32g; Net Carbs 3.5g; Protein 19g

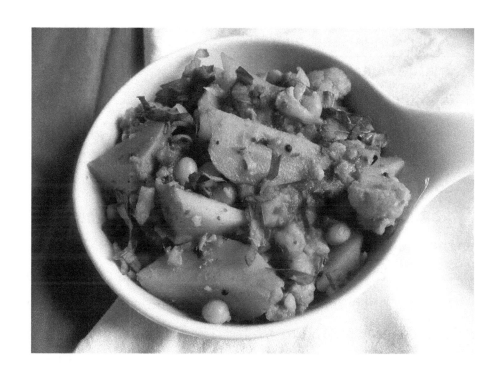

# Beef Fajitas with Colorful Bell Peppers
## Ingredients for 4 servings

1 cup mixed bell peppers, chopped

2 tbsp olive oil

2 lb skirt steak, cut in halves

2 tbsp Cajun seasoning

2 large white onion, chopped

¼ cup cheddar cheese, grated

12 low carb tortillas

**Directions and Total Time: approx. 35 min + cooling time**

Rub the steak with Cajun seasoning and marinate in the fridge for one hour. Preheat grill to 400 F.

Cook the steak on the grill for 6 minutes on each side, flipping once until lightly browned. Remove from heat and cover with foil to sit for 10 minutes before slicing. Heat the olive oil in a skillet over medium heat and sauté the onion and bell peppers for 5 minutes or until soft. Cut steak against the grain into strips and share on the tortillas. Top with the veggies and cheese and serve.

**Per serving:** Cal 512; Fat 32g; Net Carbs 4g; Protein 25g

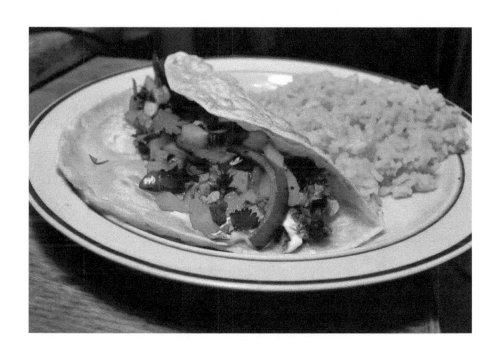

# Sweet BBQ Rib Steak

## Ingredients for 4 servings

2 tbsp avocado oil

1 ½ lb rib steaks

3 tbsp maple syrup, sugar-free

3 tbsp barbecue dry rub

**Directions and Total Time: approx. 2 hours 40 minutes**

Preheat the oven to 300 F. Remove the membrane from the steaks. Line a baking sheet with aluminum foil.

In a bowl, mix avocado oil and maple syrup and brush the mixture onto the meat. Sprinkle BBQ rub all over the ribs. Put them on the baking sheet and bake until the meat is tender and crispy on the top, 2 ½ hours. Serve with buttered broccoli and green beans.

**Per serving:** Cal 487; Net Carbs 1.8g; Fat 26g; Protein 51g

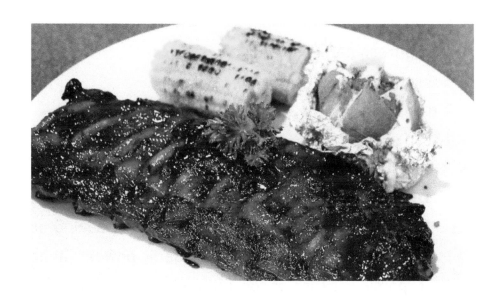

# Juicy Beef Meatballs
## Ingredients for 4 servings

1 lb ground beef

Salt and black pepper to taste

½ tsp garlic powder

1 ¼ tbsp coconut aminos

1 cup beef stock

¾ cup almond flour

1 tbsp fresh parsley, chopped

1 onion, sliced

2 tbsp butter

1 tbsp olive oil

¼ cup sour cream

## Directions and Total Time: approx. 30 minutes

Preheat the oven to 390 F and grease a baking dish. In a bowl, combine beef with salt, garlic powder, almond flour, parsley, 1 tbsp of coconut aminos, black pepper, ¼ cup of beef stock. Form patties and place on the baking sheet. Bake for 18 minutes. Set a pan with the butter and olive oil over medium heat, stir in the onion, and cook for 3 minutes. Stir in the remaining beef stock, sour cream, and remaining coconut aminos, and bring to a simmer. Adjust the seasoning with black pepper and salt.

Serve the meatballs topped with onion sauce.

**Per serving:** Cal 441; Fat 24g; Net Carbs 5.7g; Protein 31g

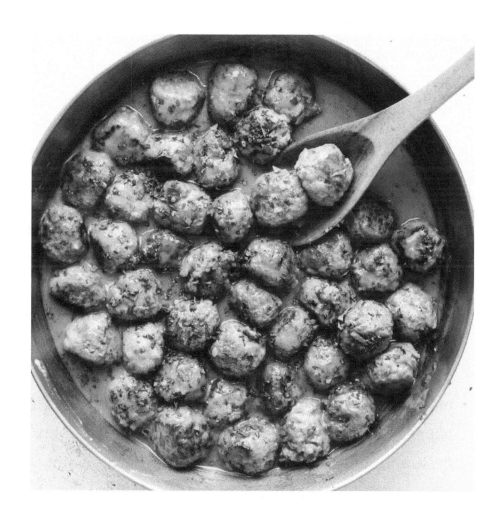

# Roasted Pumpkin Filled with Beef

## Ingredients for 4 servings

1 ½ lb pumpkin, pricked with a fork

Salt and black pepper to taste

1 garlic clove, minced

1 onion, chopped

½ cup mushrooms, sliced

28 oz canned diced tomatoes

¼ tsp cayenne pepper

½ tsp dried thyme

1 lb ground beef

1 cup cauli rice

## Directions and Total Time: approx. 70 minutes

Preheat the oven to 430 F. Lay the pumpkin on a lined baking sheet and bake in the oven for 40 minutes. Cut in half, set aside to cool, deseed, scoop out most of the flesh and let sit. Heat a greased pan over high heat. Add the garlic, mushrooms, onion, and beef and cook until the meat browns. Stir in salt, thyme, tomatoes, black pepper, and cayenne, and cook for 10 minutes; stir in flesh and cauli rice. Stuff the squash halves with beef mixture, and bake in the oven for 10 minutes.

**Per serving:** Cal 422; Fat 20g; Net Carbs 9.8g; Protein 33g

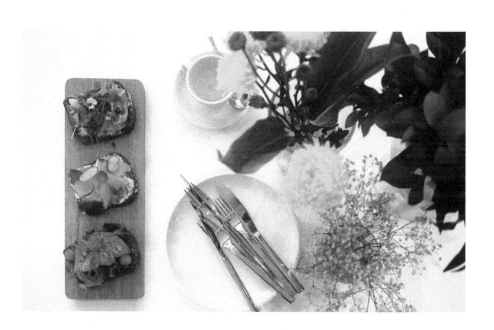

# Beef Patties with Broccoli Mash
## Ingredients for 4 servings

1 lb broccoli

1 lb ground beef

1 egg

½ white onion, chopped

2 tbsp olive oil

5 tbsp butter, softened

2 oz grated Parmesan

2 tbsp lemon juice

Salt and black pepper to taste

## Directions and Total Time: approx. 30 minutes

In a bowl, add ground beef, egg, onion, salt, and pepper. Mix and mold out 6-8 cakes out of the mixture. Warm olive oil in a skillet and fry the patties for 6-8 minutes on both sides. Remove to a plate. Pour lightly salted water into a pot over medium heat, bring to a boil, and add broccoli. Cook until tender but not too soft, 6-8 minutes. Drain and transfer to a bowl. Add in 2 tbsp of butter, and Parmesan cheese. Use an immersion blender to puree the ingredients until smooth and creamy; set aside. To make the lemon butter, mix remaining the butter with lemon juice, salt, and pepper in a bowl. Serve the cakes with broccoli mash and lemon butter.

**Per serving:** Cal 857; Net Carbs 6g; Fat 81g; Protein 35g

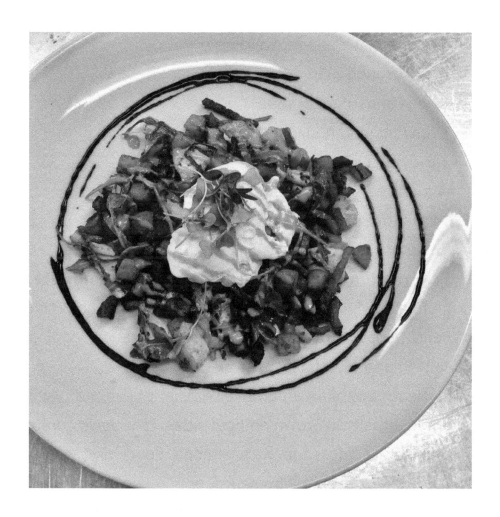

# Cocktail Chili Beef Meatballs
## Ingredients for 4 servings

2 tbsp olive oil

2 tbsp thyme

½ cup pork rinds, crushed

1 egg

Salt and black pepper to taste

1½ lb ground beef

10 oz canned onion soup

1 tbsp almond flour

2 tbsp chili sauce

¼ cup free-sugar ketchup

3 tsp Worcestershire sauce

½ tsp dry mustard

## Directions and Total Time: approx. 35 minutes

In a bowl, combine 1/3 cup of the onion soup with the beef, pepper, thyme, pork rinds, chili sauce, egg, and salt. Shape meatballs from the beef mixture.

Heat olive oil in a pan over medium heat and place in the meatballs to brown on both sides. In a bowl, combine the rest of the soup with almond flour, dry mustard, ketchup, Worcestershire sauce, and ¼ cup of water. Pour over the beef meatballs and cook for 20 minutes. Serve.

**Per serving:** Cal 341; Fat 21g; Net Carbs 5.6g; Protein 23g

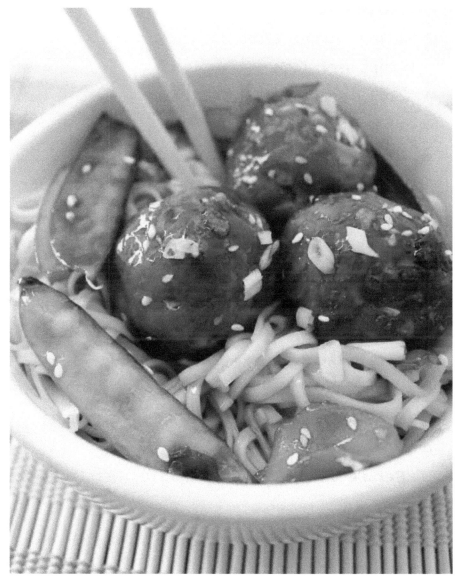

# Beef Roast with Serrano Pepper Gravy

## Ingredients for 4 servings

2 lb beef roast

1 cup mushrooms, sliced

1 ½ cups beef stock

1 oz onion soup mix

½ cup basil dressing

2 serrano peppers, shredded

**Directions and Total Time: approx. 1 hour 25 minutes**

Preheat the oven to 350 F. In a bowl, combine the stock with the basil dressing and onion soup mixture. Place the beef roast in a pan, stir in the stock mixture, mushrooms, and serrano peppers; cover with aluminum foil. Set in the oven and bake for 1 hour. Take out the foil and continue baking for 15 minutes. Allow the roast to cool, then slice, and serve alongside a topping of the gravy.

**Per serving:** Cal 722; Fat 51g; Net Carbs 5.1g; Protein 71g

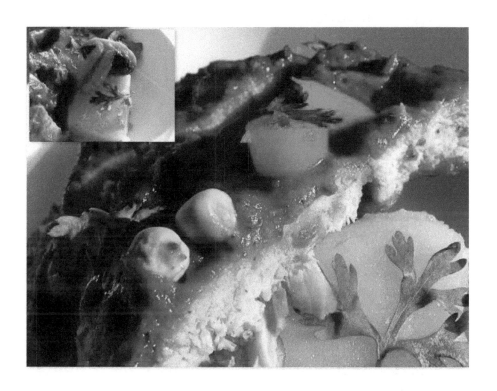

# BBQ Beef Sliders

## Ingredients for 4 servings

3 lb chuck roast, boneless

1 tsp onion powder

2 tsp garlic powder

1 tbsp smoked paprika

2 tbsp tomato paste

¼ cup white vinegar

2 tbsp tamari sauce

½ cup bone broth

¼ cup melted butter

4 zero carb buns, halved

Salt and black pepper to taste

¼ cup baby spinach

4 slices cheddar cheese

**Directions** and **Total Time: approx. 4 hours 15 minutes**

In a small bowl, combine salt, pepper, onion and garlic powders, and paprika. Cut the beef into two pieces. Rub the mixture onto the beef and place it in a slow cooker. In another bowl, mix tomato paste, vinegar, tamari sauce, broth, and melted butter. Pour over the beef and cook for 4 hours on High. When the beef cooks, shred it using two forks. Divide the spinach between buns, spoon the meat on top, and add a cheddar cheese slice. Serve.

**Per serving:** Cal 651; Net Carbs 16g; Fat 31g; Protein 69g

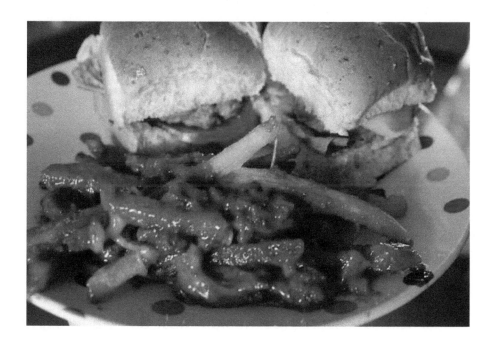

# Thyme Beef & Bacon Casserole

## Ingredients for 4 servings

2 tbsp olive oil

2 tbsp ghee

1 cup pumpkin, chopped

½ cup celery, chopped

3 slices bacon, chopped

1 lb beef meat for stew, cubed

1 garlic clove, minced

1 onion, chopped

1 tbsp red vinegar

2 cups beef stock

1 tbsp tomato puree

1 cinnamon stick

1 lemon peel strip

3 thyme sprigs, chopped

Salt and black pepper to taste

## Directions and Total Time: approx. 40 minutes

Put a saucepan over medium heat and warm oil, add in the celery, garlic, and onion and cook for 3 minutes. Stir in the beef and bacon, and cook until slightly brown. Pour in vinegar, ghee, lemon peel strip, stock, tomato puree, cinnamon stick and pumpkin. Cover and cook for

25 minutes. Get rid of the lemon peel and cinnamon stick. Adjust the seasoning and top with thyme to serve.

**Per serving:** Cal 552; Fat 41g; Net Carbs 4.5g; Protein 32g

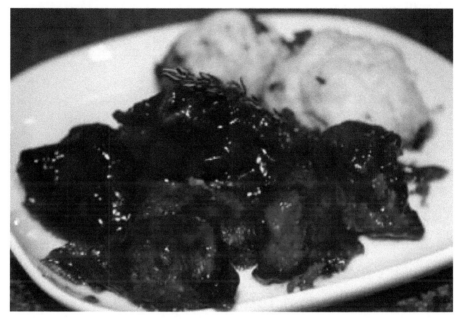

# Ground Beef Stew with Majoram & Basil
## Ingredients for 4 servings

2 tbsp olive oil

¼ cup red wine

1 lb ground beef

1 onion, chopped

2 garlic cloves, minced

14 oz canned diced tomatoes

1 tbsp dried basil

1 tbsp dried marjoram

Salt and black pepper to taste

2 carrots, sliced

2 celery stalks, chopped

1 cup vegetable broth

### Directions and Total Time: approx. 30 minutes

Put a pan over medium heat, add in the olive oil, onion, carrots, celery, and garlic, and sauté for 5 minutes. Place in the beef and cook for 6 minutes. Stir in the tomatoes, red wine, vegetable broth, black pepper, marjoram, basil, and salt, and simmer for 15 minutes. Serve and enjoy!

**Per serving:** Cal 274; Fat 14g; Net Carbs 6.2g; Protein 29g

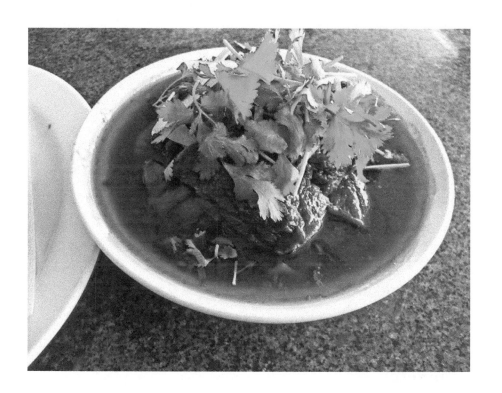

# Tomato Beef Tart with Cheddar & Ricotta
## Ingredients for 4 servings

1 egg

1 lb ground beef

2 tbsp olive oil

1 small brown onion, chopped

1 garlic clove, finely chopped

1 tbsp Italian mixed herbs

4 tbsp tomato paste

4 tbsp coconut flour

¾ cup almond flour

4 tbsp flaxseeds

1 tsp baking powder

3 tbsp coconut oil, melted

¼ cup ricotta, crumbled

¼ cup cheddar, shredded

**Directions and Total Time: approx. 1 hour 30 minutes**

Preheat oven to 360 F. Line a pie dish with parchment paper. Heat olive oil in a large skillet over medium heat and sauté onion and garlic until softened, 3 minutes. Add in beef and cook until brown. Season with herbs and stir in tomato paste and ½ cup water; reduce the heat to low. Simmer for 20 minutes; set aside.

In a food processor, add the flours, flaxseeds, baking powder, coconut oil, egg, and 4 tbsp water. Mix starting on low speed to medium until evenly combined and dough is formed. Spread the dough in the pie pan and bake for 12 minutes. Remove and spread the meat filling on top. Scatter with ricotta and cheddar cheeses. Bake until the cheeses melt and are golden brown on top, 35 minutes. Remove the pie, let cool for 3 minutes, slice, and serve with green salad and garlic vinaigrette.

**Per serving:** Cal 598; Net Carbs 2.3g; Fat 42g; Protein 61g

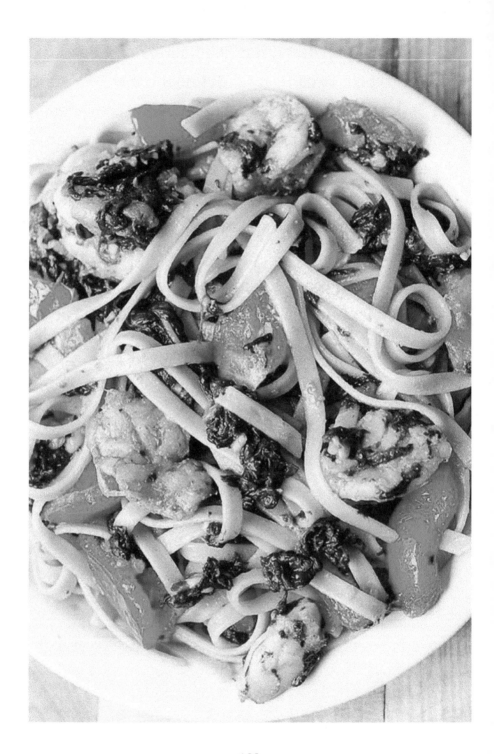

# Red Cabbage Tilapia Taco Bowl

Preparation Time **: 10 minutes**

**Cooking time** : 15 minutes

Servings **: 6**

Ingredients

- 2 cups cauli rice
- 2 tsp ghee
- 4 tilapia fillets, cut into cubes
- ¼ tsp taco seasoning
- Salt and chili pepper to taste
- ¼ head red cabbage, shredded
- **1 ripe avocado, pitted and chopped**

Directions

1. Sprinkle cauli rice in a bowl with a little water and microwave for 3 minutes. Fluff after with a fork and set aside.

2. Melt ghee in a skillet over medium heat, rub the tilapia with the taco seasoning, salt, and chili pepper, and fry until brown on all sides, for about 8 minutes in total.

3. **Transfer to a plate and set aside. In 4 serving bowls, share the cauli rice,**

**cabbage, fish, and avocado. Serve with chipotle lime sour cream dressing.**

Nutrition:

- Calories 441
- Total Fat: 12.7g
- Carbs: 71.5g
- Sugars: 2.7g
- Protein: 10.4g

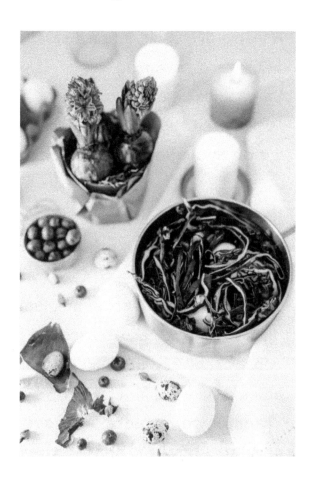

Lightning Source UK Ltd.
Milton Keynes UK
UKHW021012240621
386072UK00001B/114